Intermittent Fasting

An all-encompassing strategy for achieving sustainable
weight reduction and attaining optimalhealth
by utilizing Intermittent Fasting

*(Efficient and expedient preparation of Intermittent
Fasting dishes)*

Bernardo Hutchinson

TABLE OF CONTENT

I would like to express my gratitude for your purchase of the book titled "Intermittent Fasting: Fast & Feast: 90 Weight Loss Recipes to Eat In Between Fasts." It is my sincere hope that you will find the contents of this book both captivating and beneficial.

The global landscape is undergoing swift transformations, and failing to adapt in tandem would result in the detriment and lagging behind for individuals. It is imperative to persevere in the midst of intense competition within this fiercely competitive environment. The escalating competition has permeated nearly all facets of human existence, hence it should not be unexpected that even fundamental areas such as fitness and health have succumbed to the forces of rivalry.

Individuals universally aspire to maintain physical fitness, project aesthetic appeal, and promote overall well-being. Nevertheless, as a result of demanding schedules and an unhealthy way of life, upholding a favorable physique has become exceedingly challenging. Only a limited number of individuals possess the necessary time and resources that are paramount to cultivating our physical fitness in such a manner. While you may succeed in allocating time for physical activity, adhering to a nutritious diet continues to pose a formidable challenge. However, as a result of extensive research, the accumulated experiences, and the trials of numerous individuals grappling with a comparable predicament, a multitude of both novel and traditional dietary approaches have emerged and reemerged. These dietary regimens have greatly transformed the realm of physical fitness and have ushered in the eagerly anticipated essential transformations.

Despite the existence of numerous diets falling within the aforementioned category, one particular dietary regimen prevails significantly over all others. Intermittent fasting is a time-honored dietary approach that has experienced a resurgence in popularity due to its practicality, versatility, and numerous advantages. It is exceedingly straightforward to adhere to and yields enduring outcomes.

Intermittent fasting is a method of dietary practice that has been in existence for a significant period. Indeed, individuals have engaged in this practice since the inception of human civilization. Specific fasts like the fast observed during Ramadan and Lent, among others. have been upheld since antiquity. These rituals, founded upon deep-seated convictions and religious traditions, embody intermittent fasting practices that also yield comparable beneficial outcomes. Intermittent fasting fundamentally entails adhering to designated eating windows and abstaining from food during the remaining durations. For example, if one were to consume breakfast at 8:00 a.m., it is expected that fasting would continue until 8:00 p.m. This fasting duration provides the body with a period of rest, leading to weight reduction, regulation of glucose levels, and various other advantages.

There is a diverse range of intermittent fasting methods available. Certain tasks are straightforward for individuals at the novice level, while others pose greater difficulty. Irrespective of the relative convenience associated with intermittent fasting, undertaking this approach for individuals inexperienced with fasting can present a formidable challenge. It can be quite challenging for many individuals to establish proper regulation of their dietary cycle. However, it cannot be equated to the arduous reality of having to endure prolonged periods of hunger lasting 8-10-12 or even more hours daily. Consuming only one or two meals daily and experiencing hunger for the remainder can present notably challenging circumstances for individuals with demanding schedules, particularly those who are accustomed to eating sporadically whenever they find a moment. Individuals of this nature tend to refrain from engaging in intermittent fasting due to their conviction that they lack the ability to adhere to the prescribed dietary regimen or will experience hunger pangs as a result.

The commonly held belief that it is necessary to consume unappetizing and monotonous food during intermittent fasting is a fallacy. Numerous online resources discuss intermittent fasting, yet the vast majority neglect to acknowledge the aforementioned information. Indeed, it is entirely possible to partake in delicious yet nutritious meals during the course of intermittent fasting. To facilitate your employment, we are pleased to present a compendium of delectable nutritious recipes carefully curated to suit individuals partaking in intermittent fasting, equipped with a wide array of options for your culinary endeavors within the confines of home.

Fast & Feast – 90 Weight Loss Recipes for Consumption during Intermittent

Fasting, is a meticulously researched publication containing an extensive array of culinary options to explore during periods of fasting. These delectable culinary creations, characterized by their simplicity and expedient preparation, will yield the impeccable outcome you desire when pressed for time.

All of the recipes provided within this book have undergone rigorous testing and evaluation, ensuring their quality and reliability. Additionally, these recipes offer a significant degree of versatility. If one is dissatisfied with a particular ingredient or harbors the conviction that a recipe could be elevated with the incorporation of specific ingredients, it is possible to modify the recipe in accordance with personal preferences. Nevertheless, endeavor to preserve the nutritional composition and caloric content of the recipe.

A cookbook has the potential to greatly influence the success of a diet, and it is with complete confidence that I assure you, this particular book will unquestionably enhance your own dieting experience. I wish to express my gratitude once again for selecting this book. Now, let us commence our journey.

What Is Intermittent Fasting?

Intermittent fasting, abbreviated as IF, is a dietary practice characterized by alternating periods of eating and fasting. Its primary emphasis lies on the designated eating times, with minimal discussion concerning the requisite dietary components.

This essentially implies that it does not conform to the conventional notion of a diet, which prescribes specific foods and portion sizes. The primary focus lies in encouraging individuals to achieve a fasted state by abstaining from food for a minimum prescribed period, typically ranging from 14 to 16 hours. Subsequently, one can consume any desired food within the remaining 8 to 12 hours, contingent upon the fasting duration.

What, then, is the objective that intermittent fasting seeks to accomplish in this regard? The rationale for abstaining from food for a period of approximately 14-16 hours is to induce a state known as a fasted state. In this state, the body has completed the processes of digestion, absorption, and utilization or storage of all energy molecules derived from one's diet, namely glucose (derived from carbohydrates), fatty acids (derived from fats), and amino acids (derived from proteins). In the fasted state, your body is engaging in the active utilization of energy reserves, specifically glycogen derived from the liver and muscle cells, as well as fats obtained from diverse adipose deposits dispersed throughout the body. This entire process yields weight reduction and an extensive range of additional advantages.

I understand that you may have concerns regarding how you will manage to refrain from consuming any calorie-laden substances for a duration exceeding 14 hours. As previously stated, the actions we currently engage in are not necessarily conducive to our physical well-being. Indeed, it runs counter to the very essence of our bodies' million-year evolutionary adaptation. The concept of consuming 3 to 6 meals each day and distributing them evenly throughout the day, thereby allowing insufficient time for the body to fully metabolize the ingested food, is what is detrimentally impacting our health.

Let me explain:

Fasting Constitutes a Natural Practice

Essentially, throughout the course of history, mankind has engaged in the practice of fasting for countless generations, particularly during periods when the availability of sustenance was scarce. This is one of the factors contributing to the lower prevalence of obesity and the presence of "modern" ailments such as diabetes, obesity, neurological disorders, cardiovascular diseases, cancers, and similar conditions observed in previous times. In addition, animals possess an inherent instinct to engage in fasting periods during illness in order to expedite their healing process. Furthermore, the cyclical nature of feeding and fasting, which is customary in their natural habitat, bestows upon them the necessary energy and mental acuity to effectively hunt, even in conditions of scarce prey availability.

The crux of my argument lies in the notion that fasting is neither aberrant nor artificial; rather, our physiques possess the inherent capability to endure extended periods of abstinence from food.

Could you kindly explain the functioning principles behind intermittent fasting? Let's learn that.

The Mechanism of Intermittent Fasting

Let us commence by establishing a fundamental comprehension of the mechanisms underlying weight gain, in order to enhance our understanding of how Intermittent Fasting functions to interrupt and rectify this process.

When one consumes a conventional diet that is abundant in carbohydrates (referring to the customary American diet adhering to the USDA food pyramid), the human body proceeds to metabolize these carbohydrates into sugars or glucose, which subsequently gets assimilated into the bloodstream for distribution to various bodily organs and tissues. The purpose of glucose is to serve as a source of energy for the entirety of the human body. If there is an abundance of sugars (glucose) due to excessive consumption of carbohydrates, they are initially metabolized into glycogen within the liver, where they are subsequently stored as glycogen molecules for future utilization. However, due to the finite capacity of glycogen stores, any surplus beyond this capacity necessitates alternative storage. This 'elsewhere' refers to the adipose tissues distributed throughout the body. In order to facilitate the storage of surplus glucose as adipose tissue, it undergoes initial conversion into fatty acids and glycerol, subsequently being transported via the bloodstream as triglycerides to the lipid depots. The complete process occurs through the facilitation of insulin, a hormone synthesized by the pancreas, which encompasses the absorption of glucose by cells and the subsequent signaling of the liver to generate glycogen, fatty acids, and glycerol. The production of insulin occurs in reaction to elevating levels of glucose, therefore, an increase in glucose intake (due to higher carbohydrate consumption) leads to an augmented production of insulin. This insulin surge aids in removing excessive glucose from the bloodstream, as prolonged presence of elevated glucose levels can prove detrimental to cellular health. Consequently, as your food intake increases, so does the secretion of insulin by your body, resulting in greater accumulation of fat, particularly in the event of frequent consumption of carbohydrates. Intermittent fasting halts the entire process of supplying glucose into the bloodstream. Additionally, this dietary approach efficiently deprives the body of glucose and insulin, thereby initiating a reversal of the metabolic processes associated with high carbohydrate consumption.

Upon initiation of the fasting process, the body tends to prioritize the utilization of glycogen reserves as its initial energy source. These reserves are enzymatically converted into glucose and subsequently released into the bloodstream to serve as a direct source of usable energy. As the supplies of these stores are depleted (during the ongoing period of fasting), the body resorts to utilizing the fat that had been previously stored in the adipose tissues to meet its needs in such critical situations. In this manner, the accumulated fat reserves that have been stored over an extended period of time are actively metabolized and utilized as a source of energy. If you are amenable to a scientific explanation, allow me to elucidate the actual process that occurs during the combustion of fat:

We have identified two processes whereby the body's dependence increases as glycogen stores are depleted:

Lipolysis involves the liberation of stored fat from adipocytes into the bloodstream via molecular compounds.

The process of oxidation occurs, wherein the cells undergo combustion of the previously stored fat.

The human body induces lipolysis by means of hormonal secretion, including epinephrine, glucagon, and growth hormone (for further information). These hormones are introduced into the circulatory system, where they target adipose cells and bind to specific receptor sites. By doing so, they liberate the fatty acids that are stored internally.

IF and Women

It is imperative to acknowledge that adipocytes display significant heterogeneity and typically exhibit limited responsiveness to hormonal stimuli. As an individual with female gender who has previously pursued weight loss, it is possible that you have observed a discrepancy in the toning of different body regions, such as the arms and upper body displaying improvement while the belly and potentially the hips exhibit minimal change. This occurrence can be attributed to the presence of two opposing types of receptors, namely beta and alpha receptors, within the fat cells.

The Receptors for Beta and Alpha Stimulation

The alpha receptors serve to inhibit the process of lipolysis, whereas the beta receptors have a contrasting effect. Hence, adipocytes possessing a substantial number of beta receptors are readily attainable for mobilization, whereas those abundant in alpha receptors present a hinderance to the fat-burning process.

The resolution to this issue can be found through the identification of a method to suppress the alpha-2 receptors while maintaining the optimal functioning of the beta-2 receptors, thus promoting effective fat oxidation and facilitating weight reduction. This is where the consequences of implementing intermittent fasting arise.

Please take into consideration that when commencing intermittent fasting, there is typically a decrease in the consumption of carbohydrate-rich foods that have a propensity to increase insulin levels. As a result, there is a decrease in insulin levels within the bloodstream, leading to a simultaneous and advantageous effect in promoting fat loss. This occurs due to the inhibitory nature of insulin, which hampers the mobilization of fat. Indeed, intermittent fasting is regarded by experts in conjunction with low carb diets as the foremost strategies for suppressing alpha-2 receptors due to their notable effectiveness in curbing insulin levels. Due to reduced insulin levels, lipolysis can be facilitated, thereby leading to the breakdown of fat into fatty acids and glycerol. Subsequently, these byproducts undergo further conversion into ketones and glucose, respectively. The process of gluconeogenesis involves the conversion of glycerol into glucose, while the fatty acids undergo ketogenesis to yield ketone bodies. Due to the process of ketogenesis, the synthesis of a ketone residue called acetoacetate occurs. Consequently, this compound undergoes conversion into two additional, more diminutive iterations of ketone bodies known as BHB (Beta-Hydroxybutyrate) and acetone. The former (which holds our greater interest) exhibits greater efficiency as a fuel source, as it serves the purpose of supplying energy to the human body, including the vital organ of the brain, following a series of additional chemical reactions. In fact, research has indicated that the utilization of BHB as an energy substrate leads to improved functionality of both the brain and body, exhibiting an approximately 70% higher efficiency compared to glucose.

Hence, the practice of intermittent fasting not only facilitates weight loss but also confers the additional benefit of promoting enhanced bodily energy levels, resulting in heightened levels of vigor, increased activity, and invigoration throughout the day.

Given the emphasis on fasting within intermittent fasting, it is essential that I provide an elucidation regarding the designated timeframes for fasting and eating, in order to ensure your understanding and adherence to the prescribed regimen.

Bean And Bulgur Burger With A Spicy Twist

- Can kidney beans
- ½ cup shredded cheese
- 2 spring onions
- 1 cup of alfalfa sprouts
- Cooking spray
- 2 tbsp breadcrumbs
- ½ cup of bulgur wheat
- 2 tbsp virgin oil
- 4 oz tomato paste
- 1 tsp chili powder
- Black pepper
- 1/3 cup low fat soured cream
- Zest and juice of 1 lime

Method

Prepare the bulgur wheat according to the provided guidelines and allow it to cool thoroughly.

Create chili oil by mixing tomato paste and chili powder with virgin oil in a small skillet until it attains a yellow hue.

Combine sour cream with lime juice and zest, add seasoning, and refrigerate.

Combine the cooked bulgur, kidney beans, breadcrumbs, cheese, and spring onions with seasoning in a blender.

Create four evenly-shaped patties with a thickness of approximately three-quarters of an inch, and carefully arrange them on a baking sheet that has been lined with aluminum foil.

Proceed to grill the patties for a duration of 5 minutes on each side, ensuring they acquire a desirable golden brown hue.

Utilize cooking spray to achieve crispiness on the upper surface.

Accompany the dish with avocado and alfalfa. Incorporate sour cream and lime according to individual preferences.

One can enhance the heartiness of this meal by opting to encase the burger within pitta bread, rolls, or ciabatta.

Do you possess an affinity for pizza, despite being cognizant of its lacking in nutritional value? Experience the satisfaction of indulging in guilt-free pizza by attempting this recipe.

Forms Of Intermittent Fasting (IF)

Intermittent Fasting (IF) has been a prevalent practice in individuals' daily lives since before comprehensive research and studies were conducted. The most rudimentary version of IF occurs when an individual falls into slumber.

For instance, to illustrate the point, let us consider a scenario where an individual's last meal comprises dinner at six pm, and subsequently retiring to bed at seven pm. The following day, they arise at either six am or seven am, considering that the period of abstinence from calorie intake, known as fasting, took place during their slumber. Once more, the utilization of glycogen occurred throughout their period of sleep.

There are numerous IF methodologies accessible, contingent upon an individual's health objectives, lifestyle, and personal comfort level. Locate an option that aligns with your individual lifestyle preferences. It is important to bear in mind the significance of commencing gradually and taking measured steps when embarking upon any modification in dietary habits, as this approach facilitates long-term sustainability.

"Presented below are the two prevalent methodologies for implementing conditions:

Daily intermittent fasting can be practiced either on a daily basis or a few times per week. The objective is to enable the consumption of calories within a designated time period of four to eight hours, followed by a prescribed fasting duration, such as 12 to 24 hours.

Extended intervals of fasting are implemented on a weekly basis, usually occurring one or two times per week. The individual is permitted to follow a standard diet, followed by a cessation of calorie consumption for a duration of 24 to 32 hours (the maximum timeframe recommended by the research). The individual selects a suitable day on which they can fully unwind and remain relatively sedentary. Commence at any given hour. In the event that an individual elects to consume their final meal in the evening, specifically at six o'clock on a Friday, they are subsequently restricted to exclusively consuming water, tea, or coffee (with a preference for limiting themselves to a singular cup of coffee per day of fasting), until resuming their meals on Saturday evening at six o'clock.

Additional approaches to IF include, but are not confined to, the following:

Skipping meals is the most accessible and convenient option to commence with. The objective at hand is to deliberately select and forgo a single meal between breakfast, lunch, or dinner in a randomized manner. It could occur on a weekly basis either once or multiple times. The origins of this method can be traced back to the lifestyle of our early ancestors, who did not adhere to fixed schedules for meals or physical activity. They managed to sustain themselves with merely one or two meals per day owing to their body's utilization of stored fats as a source of energy.

The Warrior Diet prescribes a restricted eating period of four hours, followed by a fasting period of 20 hours. It is advised to refrain from consuming any food during the fasting period, although there may be some allowance for consuming small, nutritious portions of fruits or vegetables.

Variances exist in the methodologies employed, however, the shared objective among the majority of intermittent fasting techniques is to extend the duration of fasting (ranging from 12 to 32 hours) and condense the eating window to a period of four to 12 hours. An essential consideration to be mindful of during the practice of intermittent fasting is that the dietary intake within the designated "eating time frame" should primarily comprise wholesome options, avoiding processed food entirely whenever feasible, in order to optimize outcomes.

There are adverse consequences associated with unrestricted consumption of food. This may serve as a contradiction to the intended objective of intermittent fasting, as the individual may inadvertently engage in excessive consumption and compromise the efforts made towards self-discipline and abstinence.

Chapter 2: An Exposition on the Inaccuracies of Common Beliefs Regarding Weight Loss

You aspire to achieve a healthier body composition. You find yourself weary of initiating a new dietary regimen, only to subsequently revert back to your former patterns and habits. You have grown weary of consistently purchasing clothing that is one size bigger. You possess a pair of outdated denim trousers residing within your wardrobe, ostensibly serving as a source of inspiration that elicits profound antipathy within you. You are seeking a solution and a pragmatic strategy for achieving weight loss and long-term weight management. Does any of this resonate with your circumstances? How about this:

You hold the belief that eliminating your preferred culinary choices is necessary in order to achieve weight loss. It is your belief that in order to achieve weight loss, it is necessary to engage in physical exercise for a duration of at least one hour on a daily basis. You perceive that in order to shed pounds, it is necessary to abstain from consuming bread, pizza, and wine, whilst opting for salad as the principal component of each meal. You believe that in order to achieve weight loss, it is imperative to meticulously monitor and quantify caloric, carbohydrate, fat, and sodium intake for every single food item consumed.

Subsequently, mathematical computations are employed to determine one's fitness levels, which are then countered by allocating a specific duration for gym sessions, as ascertained from the aforementioned daily metrics. It is believed that in order to achieve weight loss, one must adhere to a precise daily caloric intake and caloric expenditure. Does any of that align with your comprehension of weight loss?

Nevertheless, have you made attempts at various dietary regimens only to experience disappointment and a subsequent resurgence of weight, leading to further weight gain? Alternatively, have you made attempts to enhance your exercise regimen, only to encounter excessive fatigue, physical discomfort, or excessive mental strain? The majority of the guidance currently available is impractical for individuals to consistently implement over an extended duration. Moreover, even if one adheres to certain diet regimens or exercise routines consistently, are there still specific problem areas that exhibit resistance to the notion of shrinking, becoming leaner, and losing adipose tissue? Individuals often discuss their desire to shed an additional ten pounds or the presence of persistent weight that shows resistance to reduction. This occurs due to the deliberate retention of energy by your body for purposes of "survival," as it remains under the primitive assumption that you may require this energy when evading a sabertooth tiger or enduring prolonged periods without sustenance during hunting expeditions. Your cellular composition fails to comprehend the perpetual availability of sustenance within your grasp round the clock, every single day of the year.

Fasting enables the body to rely on its reserves and eliminate them. Fasting signals the body to tap into those resilient adipose deposits and utilize their energy reserves to support bodily functions. This is the reason individuals who engage in fasting can efficiently lose weight and target the areas that appear to retain some residual weight. An additional advantage lies in the fact that this is an innate physiological process of the human body. You are not merely experiencing weight loss but concurrently promoting your overall health and welfare. If you desire to refresh your memory regarding numerous health advantages of fasting, I would recommend revisiting the initial chapter.

Naturally, this weight reduction approach is effective solely if there is excess weight that can be shed. If you find yourself exceeding the recommended weight range for your specific height and age, this solution will prove to be highly suitable and effective for you. Fasting will effectively facilitate weight loss within your body, yet it will not lead to further reduction beyond your target weight range unless intentional measures are taken to achieve such outcomes. Should you compel your body to exceed the requisite weight loss, you effectively impede your inherent mechanisms such as autophagy, consequently causing more detriment than benefit. And you will also commence to regain weight. This implies that fasting is utilized as a means to achieve an optimal and balanced weight suitable for one's body structure and age, as opposed to reducing it. The primary emphasis of fasting as a dietary practice pertains to attaining a favorable body weight rather than striving for an exceedingly thin physique. When you achieve a healthy weight range, it promotes and facilitates the internal healing and repairing mechanisms within your body. There exists a wide array of fasting regimens that one can adhere to. A comprehensive elucidation of these concepts will be provided later within the contents of this book. However, as a general principle, it can be asserted that adhering to most fasting regimens shall yield the desired outcome of attaining a healthy weight range.

Fasting elicits a notably positive response among women. The rate of response is expedited and exhibits a pronounced impact, which is equally efficacious for individuals of the male gender. In a recent research endeavor undertaken by scholars at the University of Florida, it was discovered that individuals who observed complete fasting for alternating days experienced noteworthy reductions in weight when compared to their non-fasting counterparts. The research was duplicated on ten separate occasions, and without exception, the outcomes remained consistent. While the observed reduction in body weight was substantial, the research findings also unveiled additional noteworthy advantages to their overall welfare in conjunction with the weight loss.

One notable health advantage identified pertained to the facilitation and enhancement of the individual's metabolic functioning. This phenomenon occurs due to the transition in your body's metabolism from metabolizing glucose obtained from food towards utilizing the stored fat reserves within your body. Glucose exclusively originates from dietary sources, hence rendering it addictive to the physiological processes of the body. This is also the underlying factor behind the occurrence of blood sugar crashes when one abstains from consuming carbohydrates for an extended period, as well as the subsequent surge in energy levels immediately after carbohydrate intake. Nevertheless, once the metabolic transition from glucose to fat as an energy source occurs, the body procures a fuel supply that enables a more pure and efficient combustion process. Adipose tissue undergoes the process of conversion into ketones, facilitating the strategic targeting of deep fat depots without compromising muscular integrity. When your body is engaging in the utilization of adipose tissue as an energy source, you are essentially relinquishing the retention of incoming fat and actively depleting it. Food serves its authentic function as a source of sustenance. It is no longer merely present as a contingency for situations involving a potential bear encounter or scarcity of food supplies over a limited duration. This indicates that you are engaging in the process of fat burning while simultaneously maintaining the attained results.

The human body is naturally adapted to derive its energy primarily from fatty acids and ketones. At its most fundamental level, it is inherently designed to function in this state in order to promote equilibrium and optimize overall well-being. When you engage in these practices for the betterment of your physique, you will reap manifold advantages such as reduction in body weight, improved skin complexion, enhanced cognitive focus, diminished susceptibility to a range of ailments, bolstered immune system, and additional positive outcomes. By allowing your body sufficient time, you facilitate the targeted repair, removal, and regeneration of cells, thereby ensuring the support of vital organs and tissues.

In contemporary weight-loss contexts, the term "lifestyle" is commonly employed instead of "diet". This implies that enduring modifications to your conduct must be made in order to both utilize and reap prolonged outcomes. Even diets labeled as temporary trends are attempting to assert themselves as overarching lifestyle choices. However, it is impractical to believe that one can sustain themselves solely on cabbage soup indefinitely or meticulously monitor every morsel of food consumed and subsequently determine the precise amount of time required at the gym to burn those calories. The majority of individuals do not possess ample time in their daily schedules to dedicate multiple hours towards intense physical workouts at a fitness facility in order to maintain a slim physique. Nevertheless, abstaining from food can be regarded as a genuine way of life. In order to achieve ketosis, a metabolic state characterized by the transition from glucose metabolism to the production and utilization of ketones, it is imperative to maintain unwavering adherence to your fasting regimen. Furthermore, as your overall health improves, you will experience a corresponding reduction in body weight. This phenomenon occurs due to the fact that, as time elapses, your optimal body weight undergoes a shift and is no longer congruent with the initial level at which you began. Your bodily tissues undergo a state of improved health, your physical well-being is restored, and the accumulation of adipose deposits ceases. This enables you to shed some additional weight; however, the desired outcome will not be achieved if you do not maintain regularity in your fasting.

Fad diets or alternative 'lifestyle' diet regimens prove ineffective in terms of long-term sustainability. This implies that a significant number of individuals adhering to the diet eventually revert to their former habits and experience weight gain subsequent to its conclusion. According to a statistical analysis, it was found that a majority of women, approximately over 95 percent, experienced a regression after adhering to a highly restrictive diet, thereby being unsuccessful in maintaining their weight loss in the long term. Furthermore, the participants' weight and overall well-being exhibited a decline subsequent to the completion of the dietary intervention. This location is not desirable, but rather, it is crucial to select a fasting regimen that is feasible for your circumstances, and progressively venture into more "stringent" options should you decide to do so. Further information regarding the various forms of fasting will be presented subsequently within this book. One such illustrative approach involves initiating a fasting period spanning sixteen hours on a weekly basis, progressing eventually to a duration of twenty-four hours over two or three days. This provision grants you the opportunity to select options that are environmentally conscious and genuinely compatible with your lifestyle. There is no requirement for you to effectuate any modifications at a specific moment. You have the option to implement the modifications at your convenience. Furthermore, comprehensive information regarding various fasting plans will be subsequently provided to aid you in making informed deliberations.

And during periods of non-fasting? Indeed, this eating plan presents an advantageous aspect that should be highlighted. It allows for the indulgence in all one's preferred delicacies and sustenance. This holds immense value since it eliminates the notion of personal defeat or inadequacy when partaking in a slice of birthday cake, consuming a beer during happy hour, or dining out with one's family for pizza. On days designated as non-fasting periods, one is encouraged to relish the foods of their choosing without reservation.

Nevertheless, in the event that you choose to deviate from your fasting regimen in order to indulge in culinary delights, simply reset the timer and make another attempt. It is important to recognize that this occurrence is not catastrophic in nature. This way of living can be customized to suit your individual preferences and requirements. First and foremost, it is imperative to acknowledge that achieving your weight loss objectives can be significantly facilitated and expedited by selecting nutritious foods and maintaining appropriate portion sizes during your non-restricted days. If one opts to periodically indulge in self-care rather than continuously indulging throughout non-fasting periods, the rewards will manifest more promptly. Rather than harboring the belief that you will forever be deprived of the opportunity to consume a donut, consider the notion that you may partake in indulging in one come tomorrow morning, albeit not at this precise moment. It is probable that tomorrow, either you will not remember the donut, or you will derive immense pleasure from relishing the treat that you patiently anticipated.

There are strategies that some fasting practitioners employ to expedite their progress. If you are interested in pursuing this, please take into consideration the option of incorporating a fasting-mimicking diet alongside your fasting regimen to maintain a state of ketosis within your body. The diet known as the Ketogenic diet is designed to replicate the physiological effects of fasting. This diet program adheres to a high-fat, moderate-to-low-protein, and low-to-no-carbohydrate approach. By engaging in this activity, one transitions from a condition of scarcity to a condition of ample nourishment. This stimulates and enhances your internal response mechanisms to bolster your body's functionality and facilitate weight loss more effectively. There are no prescribed guidelines dictating the manner and frequency with which the internal response system should be stimulated through fasting. The outcome will be contingent upon the characteristics of your physique and the manner in which you lead your life. Certain studies propose implementing a sixteen-hour intermittent fasting regime for a minimum of three days weekly, whereas alternative approaches advocate engaging in a 24-hour fasting period. Others adhere to a distinct amalgamation of abstaining from food, consuming nourishment, and obtaining repose. Furthermore, it is possible to maintain a consistent set of fasting days each week, or alternatively, vary them based on your personal scheduling and requirements. An alternative approach that may better accommodate your availability is to consider incorporating one or two days of fasting per week, and three days on a separate week.

The following dietary regimen serves as a recommendation for achieving rapid weight loss, sustaining the outcome, and avoiding feelings of deprivation pertaining to food or indulgences. To initiate the plan, kindly refer to your calendar and designate three days in the forthcoming week that you can regard as your "periods of reduced activity." This refers to designated days of fasting or "restriction", intended to induce ketosis and autophagy. The remaining four days of the week are designated as your "days of greater productivity or importance." Presently, these days will impede your autophagy process and disrupt your state of ketosis. A significant advantage of this strategy lies in the fact that the vast majority of your fasting period takes place during the nighttime hours. It is recommended to refrain from consuming food after a specific time in the evening prior to going to bed, ensure a minimum of eight hours of sleep, and then abstain from eating until lunchtime. Alternatively, you have the option to engage in a fasting period lasting approximately sixteen hours. The remaining eight hours of the day are allocated for the consumption of meals with minimal protein content. One can consume a wide variety of foods, but it is advised to limit carbohydrate consumption and maintain protein intake below 25 grams within that designated period. Once the 24-hour period of the "low" day has elapsed, you transition into a "high" day characterized by the absence of any limitations.

This comprehensive program has been meticulously crafted to expedite weight loss, stimulate your internal mechanisms, and provide a viable long-term strategy that can be sustained. By means of this design, you are inducing and eliciting inherent cellular and biological mechanisms within your body that enable you to attain and maintain an optimal state of health. This strategy has been devised with the intention of providing your body with essential nutrients, while also maximizing the advantages of fasting, ketosis, autophagy, and various other mechanisms.

Blueberry Cream Cheese Bombs

Ingredient List:

- Coconut cream (.25 cup)
- Softened cream cheese (4 oz.)
- Sweetener of choice
- Scant blueberries (1 cup)
- Coconut oil (.75 cup)
- Butter (1 stick)

Prep Technique:

Place a quantity of three to four berries evenly into each individual mold cup.

Gently heat the coconut oil and butter over the lowest temperature setting on the stovetop until they become liquid. Allow the mixture to reach a slightly lower temperature for a duration of approximately five minutes.

Blend together all the ingredients thoroughly using a whisk. Slowly, add the sweetener.

Using a spouted pitcher, proceed to fill an ice tray with 24 ice cubes.

Pop them out and eat when hunger strikes.

Overweight Phenomenon

Intermittent fasting offers a myriad of advantages to individuals who are affected by obesity, overweight, or possess a body mass index within the normal range. Nevertheless, it is unsuitable for certain individuals, such as pregnant and lactating women, as well as those with eating disorders and specific medical conditions.

This serves as the primary justification for your need to initiate the study of fasting's impacts on your body promptly. Pay attention to the signals your own body is sending. In the event that you observe any unwelcome secondary effects, ascertain whether they stem from mere bodily adaptation to the regimen or indicate underlying medical complications. Should you have any significant concerns regarding potential adverse effects, it is advisable to seek guidance from a medical professional in order to ensure your well-being.

What Is Obesity?

If an individual's body possesses an excess of adipose tissue that surpasses the healthy parameters designated for their specific age and gender, they can be categorized as meeting the criteria for obesity. Obesity arises as a result of an atypical or surplus accumulation of adipose tissue, commonly referred to as body fat.

A fat cell functions as an endocrine cell, constituting a hormonal component of the body, while adipose tissue serves as an endocrine organ. Comprehensive scientific investigations have substantiated the presence of excessive adipose tissue in the body, resulting in the generation of various detrimental substances, referred to as metabolites or cytokines. These substances exert adverse effects on overall health and are causally linked to the development of numerous medical complications. Adipose tissue, commonly known as fat, induces an inflammatory response, which serves as a fundamental mechanism of the body in response to infection, irritation, or any form of injury. This further emphasizes the link between increased adipose tissue in the body and the development of several disease processes. An abundance of body fat can ultimately give rise to insulin resistance, a condition wherein the hormone insulin, responsible for regulating blood sugar levels, becomes less effective. This, in turn, lays the groundwork for the onset of type 2 diabetes. How Common Is Obesity?

Obesity is widely recognized as a prevalent chronic ailment. On the other hand, there exists an urgent necessity for the establishment of fresh protocols pertaining to its healthcare prophylaxis and management.

Is my weight excessive?

One can determine if they meet the requirements for being overweight or obese by employing a straightforward mathematical equation involving their height and weight, which is known as the Body Mass Index (BMI). The figures obtained from this computation will aid you in classifying your weight, as elucidated shortly.

It is crucial to bear in mind that this numerical value may be deceiving, as it can categorize certain individuals (such as those who have a substantial amount of muscle mass or who are currently pregnant or lactating) incorrectly with regard to their actual health condition.

If your body mass index lies within the range of 18.5 and 24.9, it is determined that you possess a weight that is considered normal. Nevertheless, should your BMI be equal to or exceed 30, it can be concluded that you are afflicted with obesity, as asserted by Duerenberg et al in 1991.

The Body Mass Index (BMI) serves as the prevalent method for evaluating an individual's weight status, a tool routinely employed by medical practitioners for this purpose. Nevertheless, additional parameters such as waist circumference, waist-to-hip ratio, and various other metrics are employed as indicators of excessive adipose tissue. The measurement of waist circumference serves to ascertain the adipose tissue present in the abdominal region. An accumulation of abdominal fat, commonly referred to as "belly fat," is deemed an indicator of potential risk factors, including susceptibility to cardiovascular disease and type 2 diabetes.

Now, let us proceed to discuss the methodology for gauging your waist circumference. Initially, please ensure that you eliminate any articles of clothing from your waist area.

Assume a stance in which your feet are positioned at a distance equal to the width of your shoulders, while ensuring that your posture maintains a straight alignment of your back.

Inhale and exhale twice in a regular manner. When releasing the second exhalation, adjust the tape measure to be comfortably snug around the body without causing any discomfort or indentation.

Obtain the measurement of your waist.

Now, the complexity of these steps may appear quite daunting. An extremely straightforward and precise method for determining waist circumference entails measuring around the abdominal region at the level of the belly button or navel. This particular site frequently encompasses the broadest perimeter and is intimately linked to the vulnerability of developing metabolic disorders, such as type 2 diabetes and cardiovascular ailments.

What are the underlying reasons for my ongoing weight gain?

The human body establishes a self-determined goal or equilibrium referred to as the set point for adipose tissue (Schwartz et al., 2000). Fat serves as the primary energy source for our bodies, akin to the body's main fuel reservoir. There exist intricate signals and mechanisms that govern the quantity of adipose tissue stored within one's body. Regrettably, we possess limited dominion over the levels of adipose tissue and it is widely assumed in society that we possess the ability to consciously regulate this equilibrium.

What factors contribute to my challenges in achieving weight loss?

There persists a widespread belief among the populace that obesity can be attributed solely to the consumption of excessive calories coupled with insufficient physical activity. Regrettably, that is a misconceived notion. The concept of weight regulation bears resemblance to that of water balance regulation within the human body. In the event that you require hydration, your cerebral cortex triggers the sensation of thirst, prompting you to consume fluids. If one consumes an excessive amount of liquid, the body will eliminate the surplus water. The situation is analogous when it comes to calories and body fat. By practicing dietary restraint for a limited duration, you can exert influence over it, potentially resulting in weight reduction.

Can I Lose Weight?

The initial phase of the weight loss process involves the identification of the primary causative elements responsible for inducing obesity, which may differ from individual to individual. There is no universal or standardized solution for every situation. This occurs due to the presence of various forms of obesity, thereby necessitating the utilization of multiple therapeutic modalities and combinations thereof to facilitate the attainment of a favorable body mass among diverse individuals. Some individuals might respond favorably to modifications in their dietary practices, whereas for others, enhancing their sleep habits could lead to weight loss. It would be unrealistic to anticipate that there exists an uncomplicated resolution to attaining and sustaining a favorable body weight. It is imperative to recognize that obesity stems from diverse biological and physiological disturbances in individuals, necessitating the personalized tailoring of treatment strategies to achieve their optimal weight, utilizing a range of interventions. By implementing this approach, the odds of attaining favorable outcomes and consequently shedding excess weight are highly probable. While interventions such as engaging in regular physical activity, following a nutritious diet, implementing strategies to manage stress, and establishing healthy sleeping habits are fundamental to attaining and sustaining a healthy body weight, certain individuals may necessitate more aggressive interventions, including medical or surgical procedures, to successfully achieve weight loss. There exists a plethora of medical interventions at one's disposal for the management of obesity (Apovian et al, 2015). It is advised that you seek consultation with your healthcare provider in order to obtain a suitable referral to a medical professional specialized in the field of obesity medicine. This practitioner will conduct an in-depth interview and perform a comprehensive physical examination to determine the most suitable course of treatment in your case. In summation, given the intricate nature of obesity as a medical condition, it frequently necessitates the implementation of multiple approaches in order to attain the desired outcome of weight reduction.

Can Obesity Be Prevented?

In light of the prevailing issue of obesity, governmental officials and national organizations are examining multiple approaches and formulating strategies to cultivate an environment conducive to promoting a well-balanced lifestyle and, by extension, mitigating the prevalence of obesity. Nonetheless, given the intricate and multifaceted origins of obesity, it continues to persist as a matter of public health concern.

What is the Mechanism of Fat Processing and Storage in the Human Body?

The primary coordination of body weight and adipose tissue regulation seems to emanate from the cerebral center. The hypothalamus, situated within our brain, receives information from various sources in our body. The brain receives information about the body's energy reserves through a hormone known as leptin (Friedman and Halaas, 1998). Additionally, the brain receives signals from various organs within the body, including the pancreas and the liver. These signals provide valuable information regarding energy requirements and the availability of nutrients for the resting energy expenditure. The brain then proceeds to communicate this vital information to the rest of the body. With regards to dietary intake, the higher brain centers receive signals pertaining to the nature, scent, flavor, and consistency of food. These signals, combined with other cues originating from different organs, guide the initiation or termination of eating behavior. In general, the hypothalamus integrates and coordinates this extensive amount of information in order to establish a fat set point, which it perceives as the body's baseline. The accumulation of adipose tissue occurs in accordance with this fundamental concept, necessitating a continual effort to sustain and reach that physiological equilibrium.

What are the usual regions for fat deposition on the human body?

There exist various types of adipose tissue within the human body, namely brown fat, white fat, subcutaneous fat (primarily localized in the hips, buttocks, and thighs), and visceral fat (predominantly found in the abdominal region). Based on one's gender, race, age, and ethnicity, there is a likelihood of different patterns of fat accumulation in various regions of the body. As an illustration, it can be observed that females have a higher propensity for fat deposition in the hip and thigh regions, while males tend to exhibit a greater tendency for fat accumulation in the abdominal area, commonly referred to as abdominal fat. Adipose tissue located in the abdominal region poses a more significant health hazard compared to the fat distribution in the hips or thighs. This results in a heightened susceptibility to insulin resistance, leading to an elevated likelihood of developing diabetes, heightened levels of total cholesterol, and a predisposition to an escalated risk of stroke and cardiovascular disease (Schneider et al., 2010).

What are the adverse health and well-being implications of being overweight?

Recent research has indicated that obesity is responsible for, or has contributed to, over 40 separate ailments that result in compromised health and a diminished standard of living (Cummings et al, 2002). The medical complexities encompass a spectrum of conditions, including metabolic disorders like type 2 diabetes mellitus and elevated cholesterol levels, as well as hypertension, gallstones, hepatic steatosis, pancreatitis, obstructive sleep apnea, and even reproductive impairments. Additional ailments frequently linked to obesity comprise of stress incontinence (characterized by the inability to regulate urination), heightened intracranial pressure (known as idiopathic intracranial hypertension), manifesting as headaches, degenerative joint disease (commonly referred to as arthritis), and spinal disc disease. Scientific inquiry has further substantiated a robust correlation between obesity and numerous forms of cancer.

Is Obesity Inherited?

Thus far, our understanding suggests that obesity is a multifaceted condition stemming from a multitude of interplays between hereditary and environmental factors. It is now widely recognized that various manifestations of obesity tend to aggregate within familial relationships. The likelihood of developing obesity is significantly higher, by a factor of two to eight, for individuals with a familial predisposition to obesity compared to those without any familial history of obesity. Additionally, the risk is even more pronounced in individuals with severe obesity (Zlot et al, 2007).

Research conducted on twins has examined individuals who were raised in the same environment versus those who were raised in dissimilar circumstances. These researchers have confirmed that the impact of genetics on body mass index (BMI) is significant (Stunkard et al., 1990).

There exist additional uncommon factors contributing to genetic obesity, where a solitary gene is impacted, resulting in more severe manifestations of obesity. These particular forms of obesity are predominantly observed during the early stages of childhood. In brief, it can be generally observed that genetic variation predominantly impacts an individual's susceptibility to obesity, yet the influence of environmental and psychological factors plays a substantial role in its manifestation. Our comprehension of the genetics that influence weight and control energy regulation is advancing swiftly.

Is there an increased propensity for weight gain as one progresses in age?

The aging process is accompanied by alterations in the composition of the physique. According to imaging studies, it has been observed that the quantity of subcutaneous fat, the adipose tissue located beneath the skin, tends to diminish while the amount of visceral fat, the adipose tissue located in the abdominal region, tends to escalate as individuals grow older. The presence of visceral fat is undesirable, as previously elucidated. It is linked to systemic inflammation, and it steadily augments the susceptibility to coronary artery disease, stroke, and mortality. In addition to the modification of body composition, a significant alteration that occurs with age entails the reduction of skeletal muscle mass. Muscular strength aids in the maintenance of a heightened metabolic rate and an elevated resting energy expenditure. Consequently, the decline of the aforementioned leads to a decrease in the overall energy outflow. The modified composition of the body and decline in muscle mass precipitates an increase in adipose tissue accumulation.

The relationship between insulin sensitivity and both the accumulation of visceral fat and the decline in muscle mass has been established. As the body's sensitivity to insulin decreases, there is an accompanying increase in the secretion of insulin. Given its role as a storage hormone, this metabolic hormone is responsible for a multitude of issues. It facilitates the enhancement of glucose absorption and the synthesis of fat, while concurrently diminishing the oxidation of fat and stored glycogen.

What measures can I take to address my surplus body weight?

There exists a variety of efficacious treatment alternatives for weight reduction. In order to determine the most appropriate course of treatment to address your specific requirements, it will be necessary to undergo a thorough evaluation conducted by a qualified physician specializing in obesity medicine. Furthermore, it is crucial to seek guidance from both a nutritionist and a psychologist. Once you have completed a comprehensive assessment, which may involve blood analysis, your physician and the entire healthcare team will collaborate with you to establish an appropriate course of action.

There are multiple treatment modalities available, encompassing behavioral, medical, and surgical approaches. Behavioral treatment encompasses implementing lifestyle adjustments, including adopting more wholesome dietary selections, integrating additional physical activity into daily routines, and ensuring the maintenance of an optimal and regular sleep regimen.

If your physician deems that lifestyle adjustments alone are not likely to yield significant benefits, particularly in cases involving a track record of consistent lifestyle modifications, severe obesity, or moderate obesity alongside multiple obesity-related comorbidities (such as hypertension, type 2 diabetes, or obstructive sleep apnea), a course of pharmacotherapy could be considered. A multitude of weight-loss medications are accessible for potential use in achieving weight reduction; nonetheless, solely a physician possesses the authority to prescribe such medications for your specific needs. Once you initiate a medication, it is necessary to undergo regular monitoring in order to evaluate the efficacy and potential adverse effects of the prescribed treatment. These medications are administered for extended periods of time, as cessation of their usage frequently results in an increase in body weight.

What is Emotional eating?

As evident to even individuals without professional expertise, healthcare professionals classify mental and physical illnesses based on a variety of criteria. These classifications encompass terms such as "disease" (for example, Lyme disease), "condition" (for example, psychological condition), and "syndrome" (for example, toxic shock syndrome); however, few individuals without specialized knowledge comprehend the nuanced differences between them. However, it is imperative to comprehend the relevance of this classification in relation to this pathological condition, as it provides elucidation on the scientific perspective of this malady and how interventions aim to address it.

Although BED is accompanied by various physical manifestations, including comorbidities, it is widely recognized as a psychological condition rather than a physical affliction, characterized as an abnormal social behavior. Consequently, the most effective approach to its management is through psychological therapy. It should be noted that while medical doctors and other therapeutic practitioners can indeed provide assistance in mitigating numerous symptoms related to binge-eating disorder, it is crucial to recognize that these approaches predominantly address the symptoms rather than the underlying cause(s) of the issue. Therefore, the initial stage in comprehending binge-eating disorder lies in recognizing that one is confronted with a consequential psychological matter, which subsequently translates into physical manifestations.

Do you experience the condition of emotional eating?

Levels of obesity among individuals are unquestionably surpassing any historical precedent. This phenomenon has permeated various regions across the globe. There is a concerning trend of individuals experiencing an unprecedented increase in weight. However, the primary inquiry remains: what is the underlying reason behind this occurrence? What is the underlying factor leading to the increase in individuals' body weight?

The immediate solution would involve attributing it to the consumption of unhealthy food, which constitutes the rational course of action. Numerous food manufacturing companies are responsible for producing unhealthy junk foods that are not conducive to the well-being of individuals.

Junk foods can be described as food products that have undergone modifications from their original composition, resulting in processed items. Processed food items commonly found in the market often contain additional substances such as pesticides, preservatives, artificial flavorings, refined sugars, excessive amounts of salt, various seasonings, and other components that have detrimental effects on our overall well-being.

Consuming artificial food products can result in experiencing an unnatural sensation. Put another way, these factors will induce sensations of stress, anxiety, agitation, erratic heart rate, and additional related symptoms.

Although these symptoms may be inherent in certain life circumstances, their occurrence solely due to food consumption renders them atypical.

The Real Reason

It is widely acknowledged that the consumption of unhealthy food is the primary contributing factor to a significant proportion of health issues prevalent in both America and other advanced nations. As long as government agencies have not instituted regulations prohibiting the sale of unhealthy food items in supermarkets, such products will continue to be available for purchase and remain in demand by consumers.

The presence of junk food in supermarkets is widely acknowledged by the general populace as detrimental to their well-being. They are aware that consuming cookies, cakes, pizza, and fried foods will inevitably induce feelings of discomfort and unease. However, they persist in consuming these food items. So again, why?

The primary contributing factor pertains predominantly to stress, more so than any other aspect. In the contemporary era, individuals lead exceedingly hectic and anxiety-inducing lifestyles. They must be concerned with securing their livelihood, attending to the welfare of their children, and similar responsibilities. It reaches a juncture where individuals are devoid of any opportunity to unwind and experience a sense of ease.

Individuals experiencing high levels of stress often develop unfavorable behavior patterns as a means to alleviate their stress. One of the most significant tendencies that individuals acquire is indulging in excessive consumption of unhealthy food.

Upon occurrence of this event, the synthetic chemicals and additives present in said food products will elevate their levels of stress to an even greater extent. Hence, rather than remedying the issue, consumption of junk food exacerbates it.

The Influence of Stress on Body Weight

Unaddressed stress serves as a notable contributor to weight gain due to its propensity to trigger emotional overeating. As an illustration, individuals commonly resort to consuming an entire container of ice cream, devoid of rational thought or emotional consideration, in an endeavor to combat stress, particularly within the confines of the workplace. In an endeavor to meet demanding work deadlines, some individuals passionately consume french fries and hamburgers while seated at their workstations. Perhaps you are a diligent mother who must transport your children to school before hurrying to work, dedicating yourself to the constant movement required to meet strict deadlines for numerous engagements and a multitude of meetings. In no time, one realizes the lack of opportunity to consume meals mindfully, consequently leading to the engagement in emotional overconsumption of cookies within the confines of one's vehicle. It is possible that as a small business owner, you may be making fervent attempts to ensure smooth operations, only to realize one day that there has been a noticeable increase in your physical girth. In the event that you are detained in any of these situations, it is important to note that you are not by yourself, and the probability remains significant that you are not responsible for this predicament. This level of pressure fosters an environment conducive to weight gain, particularly in prolonged durations. Initially, it poses a significant challenge for us to adopt a wholesome way of life owing to the detrimental impact it exerts on our determination to do so. Additionally, it amplifies our predisposition to engage in emotional eating and promotes the retention of adipose tissue, leading to its accumulation within our physiological systems.

Hence, what are the biological and psychological determinants underlying the phenomenon of overeating and subsequent weight gain in relation to stress? Allow us to examine several factors contributing to the correlation between stress and weight gain.

Effects of Stress on the Endocrine System

The body undergoes a hormonal response, characterized by the release of various hormones including cortisol, adrenaline, and CRH, when the brain detects any type of peril or imminent harm. Whether you find yourself confronting a difficult supervisor, grappling with the burden of a substantial credit card payment, or hustling to meet demanding deadlines, your brain sends signals to your body to unleash these chemicals, aiding in the management of the perceived threat. These hormones serve the purpose of priming your body and mind to confront adversity, enhancing your resilience or sharpening your vigilance for action.

In anticipation of the fight-or-flight response, adrenaline prompts the rapid movement of blood from the internal organs to the muscles, resulting in decreased anger levels. Nonetheless, the presence of cortisol, referred to as the stress hormone, endures for an extended period subsequent to the dissipation of adrenaline's impact. This hormone initiates communication with the body, prompting an increased demand for nourishment. Please be aware that your neuroendocrine system does not discriminate between the different types of threats you may encounter. Our predecessors necessitated considerable energy reserves in order to contend with untamed creatures, thus necessitating augmented storage capacities for glucose and fat within their physiques.

Nevertheless, in the present day, we find ourselves in the position of spending extended periods at our desks, diligently striving to meet stringent timeframes, or reclining on our sofas, burdened with concerns over the resolution of expenses by month's end. In contrast to our predecessors who exerted tremendous effort in confronting the specific threats and perils they encountered, the current stressors we confront do not elicit the same level of physiological response from our bodies. However, the human mind is incapable of perceiving this distinction, as it lacks the ability to register such alterations within our neuroendocrine framework. Consequently, individuals often find themselves inclined to indulge in an additional serving of cookies, hamburgers, or fries as a means to restore their body's nutrient reservoir. The brain perceives all types of stress as a potential danger and endeavors to ready the body to cope with it. You experience a propensity for excessive consumption of food, resulting in subsequent weight gain.

Associations between Stress and Abdominal Adiposity

Excessive abdominal fat and the accumulation of weight in the waist area have been specifically correlated with persistent stress. A multitude of individuals reside in a state of apprehension towards what is unfamiliar. The issue lies in the body's inability to discern between anxiety that poses a severe threat to life and stress that arises due to occupational pressures. The act of missing the train due to lateness, or the stress caused by struggling to manage financial obligations and payments, is equated with the necessity of fleeing from a structure at risk of collapsing. All of these stressors are handled in a similar manner, with the brain taking the lead in the release of adrenaline and cortisol to prime us for the instinctual response of fight or flight, much like our ancestors did when confronted with perilous encounters with tigers and lions.

Presently, the nature of the stress we encounter does not necessitate engaging in physical combat or fleeing, owing to the modern way of life, and it happens to persist without interruption.

Consequently, following periods of heightened stress experienced either in the professional realm or within personal relationships, there will be a sustained elevation in cortisol levels, thereby leading to an augmented desire for food. Your physiological system continues to interpret the need to replenish your energy reserves for glucose and fat following the strenuous exertion endured during the confrontation and escape from a stressor. Hence, when one is engaged in a demanding lifestyle, a perpetual sensation of hunger tends to prevail. One develops an inclination towards carbohydrates and fats as a result of a physiological urge to accumulate energy-rich sustenance. Consequently, in the presence of chronic stress, your body anticipates the need to engage in a response of either fighting or fleeing in order to escape potential harm or danger. Failure to do so will result in the body storing glucose and fat as adipose tissue around the abdominal region. The reason why fat tends to accumulate in the abdominal region is because of its proximity to the liver, allowing easy access to energy stores that can be readily converted when demanded. Cortisol, known as the stress hormone, has the effect of decelerating the body's metabolic processes with the purpose of supporting sufficient glucose provision to cope with the demanding physiological and cognitive strain involved in addressing your sources of stress. As a result, the amount of fat burned is insufficient, resulting in greater accumulation of abdominal fat and subsequent weight gain in the abdominal area.

Heightened levels of stress and anxiety

In the event of a threat or danger, when adrenaline triggers the fight or flight response, individuals often become physically agitated and restless. As anxiety arises, one experiences a state of heightened alertness as adrenaline reacts to the perceived stressor. One may note a prevailing sense of unease, prompting a propensity to engage in frantic activity while seeking a resolution. This level of distress elicits a response of indulging in food for comfort. In an endeavor to achieve a sense of tranquility, individuals often resort to consuming or excessively indulging in food items that are detrimental to their health. This phenomenon is a commonly observed reaction to psychological stress.

Anxiety precipitates thoughtless consumption, leading to heightened food intake without achieving a sense of satiety. Due to your preoccupation with distressing and burdensome thoughts, your capacity to discern the quantity of food consumed is hindered, thereby inhibiting your ability to fully appreciate and savor the taste of the food. When experiencing anxiety and stress, individuals tend to engage in emotional overeating and lack mindful awareness, resulting in diminished feelings of satisfaction despite increased consumption. This excessive consumption driven by emotional distress and anxiety results in an increase in body weight.

Stressful Cravings and fast food

Persistent stress is typically accompanied by a proclivity for indulging in food items that provide immediate solace, such as ice cream, hamburgers, freshly baked cookies, and potato chips. These food products are extensively processed and conveniently consumable, containing elevated quantities of sodium, glucose, or saturated fats. There are both psychological and biological factors that contribute to this intense desire. It is plausible that an alteration in the brain's reward system due to heightened stress and elevated cortisol levels could potentially trigger an increased desire for sugar and fat consumption. Furthermore, in times of stress, it is common for individuals to seek solace in nostalgic recollections from their childhood, particularly when these memories evoke a sense of comfort through the consumption of confectionery.

Due to the cognitive effort and time required to meticulously plan and prepare a nutritious meal, you find yourself incapable of accomplishing this task. It is more probable that you would commute to the fast-food establishment in order to indulge in these extensively processed food items and reward yourself accordingly. A significant proportion of individuals residing and employed in urban localities exhibit a decreased tendency to engage in the practice of preparing and consuming evening meals within their own residences. This phenomenon can be primarily attributed to the presence of traffic congestion, which consequently amplifies the stress levels experienced as one traverses from their workplace to their place of residence. You arrive home at a late hour, experiencing heightened hunger and a significant impairment of your self-control.

Your sole course of action entails operating a vehicle to the adjacent culinary establishment in order to procure sustenance for the evening meal. One tends to consume nutritionally deficient foods absentmindedly and impulsively, resulting in weight gain attributed to the substantial quantities of sodium, saturated fat, and added sugars present in such dietary choices.

Less Sleep

As per the survey conducted by the American Psychological Association (APA) titled "Stress in America," it has been determined that over 40% of the American population experiences difficulty in falling asleep due to stress. During the nighttime hours, it is possible that you may experience a state of restlessness, wherein you remain awake, contemplating concerns regarding financial obligations, work-related challenges, and the dynamics within your relationships. You harbor concerns regarding the provision of care for your children during your departure from home for occupational endeavors.

Research suggests that concern or preoccupation can be a significant factor contributing to insomnia. The cognitive faculties resist being deactivated due to excessive stimulation, thus resulting in hyperactivity. If one is a student, they may experience nights of sleeplessness as they diligently work on writing notes or preparing for their examinations. During such moments, it is possible for individuals to experience sleep disturbances as a result of the heightened psychological and physiological strain caused by such eleventh-hour pressures.

Such stress leads to fatigue as a consequence of the reduction in blood sugar levels. If one were to employ the tactic of consuming beverages containing caffeine, such as coffee, in an effort to prolong wakefulness, it would only serve to exacerbate the disruption of their sleep-wake rhythm. Other individuals turn to consuming alcoholic beverages in an attempt to alleviate their distress during such challenging circumstances, thereby exacerbating the situation.

Regarding the matter of impacting body weight loss or gain, sleep plays a consequential role. Leptin and ghrelin are the hormones responsible for the regulation of appetite, and sleep deprivation can potentially disrupt their normal functioning. In instances where you are experiencing fatigue or irritability due to insufficient sleep, it is common to develop a propensity for consuming food that contains elevated levels of sugars, particularly carbohydrates. Insufficient sleep can contribute to the erosion of one's willpower, rendering individuals more susceptible to succumbing to mindless and emotional temptations of consuming unhealthy food choices. Sleep deprivation will inevitably result in the accumulation of excess weight.

THE COMPREHENSIVE GUIDE TO INTERMITTENT FASTING AND ITS IMPACT ON WOMEN

There is considerable divergence in opinions regarding the participation of women in fasting for the purpose of weight loss or to potentially derive other health advantages. The primary underlying factor for this phenomenon stems from a series of studies conducted over the past century, which have revealed distinct divergences in the physiological responses of women's bodies to fasting compared to those of men subject to equivalent fasting durations. With the abundance of available information and extensive promotions, individuals may encounter challenges in determining whether Intermittent Fasting is suitable for their specific needs. In the following chapter, we shall delve into both the favorable aspects of Intermittent Fasting as well as the potential hazards and challenges that individuals have encountered in their fasting endeavors.

Does this imply that women ought not to refrain from fasting? Absolutely not. Women just face different challenges with fasting which means that every woman will have unique modifications they make to their Intermittent Fasting schedule. Fitness professionals, nutritionists, and medical experts universally advise women to adopt a more lenient approach to fasting than men in order to safeguard crucial female bodily functions from adverse alterations or complications.

The physiological functioning of the female body is more reliant on calorie intake and hormone balances compared to males, and both of these factors are significantly impacted upon initiation of fasting. Female individuals should bear in mind that when conducting research and devising a schedule for Intermittent

Fasting, it is advisable to commence by gradually reducing calorie intake for briefer durations, rather than immediately engaging in complete fasting on alternate days. After the body has acclimated to the alteration, it becomes possible to subsequently decrease calorie intake or prolong fasting intervals until the desired target is achieved.

The Advantages and Benefits of Implementing Intermittent Fasting

Individuals who keenly stay attentive to updates regarding the latest health trends are undoubtedly familiar with the advantages of Intermittent Fasting and its widespread appeal. There is a plethora of reviews and blog posts readily available across the internet discussing the program's personal modifications that have proven effective for individuals, as well as the subsequent success stories of fasting. Individuals of varying age brackets are extolling the virtues of Intermittent Fasting for its profound enhancements to their overall health and well-being. Moreover, they eagerly anticipate the opportunity to motivate and guide others through visual evidence of their own progress and by providing valuable recommendations.

"Several benefits can be derived from selecting Intermittent Fasting as the preferred approach for achieving weight loss goals, such as:

The aspect of convenience: Devoting time and energy towards adhering to daily dietary and exercise regimens can already be challenging, making the integration of a fasting schedule seem burdensome! A significant factor contributing to the widespread adoption of Intermittent Fasting is the absence of a need to adhere strictly to a predetermined routine. You possess the ability to customize your fasting periods to align with your current schedule, enabling you to fast at the most optimal times for your convenience.

Simplicity: Intermittent Fasting can be easily comprehended and mastered with diligent research and obtaining a thorough comprehension of its principles. After selecting your preferred timetable and optimized moments to enhance the effectiveness of your fasting endeavors, all that remains is to commence your journey. There exists neither any subscriptions nor any gym memberships. There is no need for significant expenditures on equipment, ingredients, or supplements. Many individuals who adhere to Intermittent Fasting protocols often experience financial savings in the long run due to the decrease in food purchases during their non-fasting periods, as their bodies gradually adapt to a lower daily caloric intake.

Compatibility with Different Dietary Plans: Given that the Intermittent Fasting regimen does not prescribe specific food choices, individuals already content and achieving positive outcomes with their existing diet can rest assured that they need not make any dietary adjustments. Individuals seeking to modify their dietary habits upon commencing intermittent fasting should prioritize the adoption of low-calorie, protein-rich meal plans, as these can effectively augment the weight reduction and wellness advantages associated with this fasting practice.

There is an abundance of positive information for individuals who are prepared to begin their own Intermittent Fasting regimen, including an equal number of health benefits and program advantages.

An important advantage of practicing Intermittent Fasting, which has its origins in early medical theories, is its capacity to purify and rid the body of detrimental substances and forces. After the elimination of these toxins, the body has the chance to facilitate healing of muscle and cellular degeneration, promote digestive well-being, and aid the brain in balancing sleep patterns.

Intermittent Fasting participants derive an array of additional physical advantages, such as:

Enhanced cognitive acuity and neural activity

Inducing autophagy, the biological mechanism responsible for replacing deteriorated components of cells with newly regenerated cellular material, and initiating the process of cellular purification.

Enhanced metabolic efficiency for fat oxidation

Reduce cholesterol and blood sugar levels

Reduction of systemic inflammation.

The potential to enhance overall longevity and enhance physical capabilities during the later stages of life.

Additionally, certain individuals experience a heightened development of muscular tissue when undergoing weight loss. Although this phenomenon is predominantly observed among males, females also experience advantages in terms of weight loss and muscle development through consistent adherence to Intermittent Fasting.

One of the most remarkable advantages cited by individuals who grapple with diabetic symptoms or other ailments related to blood sugar is the notable improvement in their essential health metrics facilitated by the practice of Intermittent Fasting. In addition to their medically recommended medication, individuals who engage in fasting have observed significant improvements in their body's insulin sensitivity, thereby decreasing the likelihood of developing

Type 2 diabetes. There have been instances where individuals practicing Intermittent Fasting, coupled with medical intervention, physical activity, and appropriate dietary choices, have observed a reversal of their preexisting diabetic symptoms.

Another advantage valued by adherents of the Intermittent Fasting regimen is the comprehensive nature of weight loss experienced during fasting, encompassing all regions of the body, including the central or abdominal region. The central region of the body is the primary site for the accumulation of body fat, particularly among individuals, especially women. Intermittent Fasting specifically focuses on the adipose tissue, which represents the prominent fat reserves within the human body. Consequently, individuals who encounter difficulties in shedding weight and bulk in this particular region would likely observe a decrease in said aspects once their body has undergone an adaptation to fasting.

This chart illustrates the outcomes of a three-week research study conducted on individuals who were new to practicing Intermittent Fasting. Below, you will find the measurements of the study participants and their respective progress.

Factors to Contemplate Prior to Embarking on Intermittent Fasting

Indeed, contemplating the commencement of a fasting regimen becomes invigorating as one acquaints oneself with the manifold merits or observes acquaintances and admired personalities sharing the success they have achieved through Intermittent Fasting. Nevertheless, Intermittent

Fasting necessitates utmost dedication and unwavering perseverance, as it is a significant undertaking that impacts both your mental and physical well-being. Improper execution of Intermittent Fasting can also give rise to enduring detrimental impacts on the body, which can be mitigated by vigilantly monitoring specific indicators.

The majority of these adverse effects wane as the body acclimates to the caloric modifications over time, either upon the development of a habitual fasting routine or the discontinuation of the intermittent fasting regimen (depending on whether one is commencing or concluding an Intermittent Fasting regimen). Notwithstanding the transient nature thereof, any adverse bodily manifestations experienced upon commencing the fasting regimen should not be disregarded, and it is advised to duly consult with your personal physician should they escalate in severity.

One aspect that is often overlooked by individuals prior to embarking on a fast is the enhanced effectiveness and enhanced likelihood of sustaining an Intermittent Fasting regimen when gradually transitioning into it. This holds particular significance for individuals who are fasting for the first time. Your objective may consist of practicing intermittent fasting for intervals of 18 to 24 hours on alternate days; however, such a regimen can cause significant physiological distress and psychological fatigue. If you possess no prior experience in fasting or have refrained from fasting for an extended period, it is advisable to initiate your journey with a less rigorous fasting regimen. This approach will grant your body the opportunity to acclimate and adequately ready itself for subsequent stages. By allowing your body additional time to adjust, you will mitigate the likelihood of encountering adverse consequences as you persist with your fasting regimen.

Social media platforms have enabled individuals to actively engage in the dissemination and preservation of their daily activities. This inherent desire to present ourselves prominently implies that the majority of individuals have already acclimated to capturing photographs of themselves and their experiences for the purpose of sharing them with their acquaintances. A common sentiment among individuals who have made significant advancements in their weight reduction and overall well-being is that they desire or are pleased to have captured visual documentation of their progress at frequent intervals. Progress pictures can serve as a valuable source of motivation to reaffirm your belief in and reignite your commitment to your Intermittent Fasting regimen, even if their purpose is not to be shared with others. Challenging days lie ahead, and the allure of temptation is ever present in close proximity. The greater the arsenal of resources at your disposal, the higher the likelihood of averting surrender or abandonment.

Please be advised that acquiring comprehensive knowledge about a subject is invaluable, thus I encourage you not to compromise on your research endeavors. This holds particular significance if you have perused the blog articles and engaged in conversations with individuals who are already practicing Intermittent Fasting, yet still possess reservations or apprehensions regarding your potential health prospects pertaining to fasting.

The Primal State of Affairs: Examining the Origins of Our Foundations

An obstacle encountered by women lies in situations where they experience a minor increase in weight in the aftermath of discontinuing fasting, attributed to the subsequent elevation in their overall food consumption and the restoration of their dietary patterns. This phenomenon constitutes an innate defensive reaction by which the female organism undergoes during instances of abrupt escalation in calorie intake, and can be traced back to the primitive origins of our species. Primitive human beings were hunters and gatherers who depended entirely on their surroundings for sustenance. Deprived of any form of refrigeration or preservation, their sustenance comprised solely of what was necessary, leaving them uncertain about the source of their next meal. During periods of food scarcity, they would engage in fasting regimes, during which their bodies would adapt to functioning with a reduced caloric intake. The human body, in the face of uncertain caloric availability and its imperative need for energy, underwent an adaptation wherein a substantial portion of the ingested calories were stored within adipose tissue, resulting in a physiological phenomenon commonly referred to as "water weight."

Genetic researchers posit that it is during this particular period that the human body underwent the evolutionary modifications in genetics and hormonal regulation observed in contemporary Homo sapiens. Hence, women may experience a marginal increase in weight during the initial days subsequent to an extended period of practicing Intermittent Fasting. After adapting to varying levels of food intake, the female physique efficiently utilizes the surplus calories it receives upon cessation of fasting, subsequently storing them for future energy requirements. It's an instinctual, unconscious response that roots into our very nature as human beings.

Not all females undergo this initial gain in weight, however, for those who do, there are strategies available to counteract it. The positive aspect regarding water weight is that once the body acclimates to the heightened caloric consumption, that weight will subsequently diminish.

Women who partake in fasting can also mitigate or eradicate this concern by progressively reducing their Intermittent Fasting routine as they deem fit to conclude it. For individuals who fully abstain from consuming food throughout fasting intervals, we recommend gradually concluding their fasting process by following these steps. Please bear in mind the importance of allowing your body an appropriate period to acclimate to each phase prior to progressing further.

1. Reduce the duration of fasting and refrain from augmenting caloric intake by resuming the habitual or nearly equivalent calorie consumption during non-fasting periods. For instance,

consider distributing your eating periods throughout any additional available time, opting for smaller, lower calorie meals consumed at shorter intervals, rather than consuming one or two large meals prior to fasting once more.

2. Gradually augment your calorie intake by 25% of your daily caloric consumption biweekly throughout the fasting periods. Continue this practice until you have achieved a balance in caloric intake between former fasting days and eating days, resulting in the normalization of your diet.

3. In the event that you observe a rise in your weight during any phase of the plan, gradually augment your physical activity until the apparent retention of

water diminishes. This can be achieved by modestly amplifying the intensity of your workout, extending the duration of your routine by thirty minutes, incorporating an additional lap around your surroundings, or alternatively, opting for staircases whenever available to facilitate the expenditure of the surplus calories retained by your body.

Please be reminded that these steps should be considered as suggestions, and it is possible to modify your plan according to your body's reaction to caloric changes, in the event that you decide to discontinue fasting. Please consult your healthcare provider if you have any inquiries regarding additional fasting choices and personalized modifications to your program.

Confirmed Strategies For Alleviating Appetite During Intermittent Fasting

1. Maintain Proper Ratios of Macronutrients such as Protein, Carbohydrates, and Fats

Many individuals struggle with intermittent fasting primarily because they adopt an excessively low carbohydrate approach, consequently repeatedly inducing a state of ketosis. This can prove highly detrimental for brief periods of intense physical exertion.

Carbohydrates: The recommended minimum intake is 0.6g per pound of body mass to maintain a state of non-ketosis.

Certain individuals may also experience enhanced satiety when consuming higher amounts of carbohydrates.

It is advisable to maintain fat intake within the range of 25-30% of total calorie consumption.

2. Do not confuse hunger with dehydration.

Hunger cues can frequently be deceptive - typically, our bodies simply require hydration.

In order to ensure proper hydration, it is recommended to carry a reusable bottle with you and strive to consume one gallon of water daily.

3. Tea and coffee have tremendous benefits.

Consuming coffee and tea can effectively alleviate hunger pangs during a fasting period. Prior to delving into the methodology of the matter, it is imperative to elucidate the types of coffee and tea that can be ingested without infringing upon the observance of fasting. When considering coffee, it is important to note that any type of black coffee will not disrupt the fasting period.

Black coffee contains no creamers, milk, or sugar.

If you have a strong aversion to black coffee and desire a sweet flavor, it is possible to incorporate small quantities of a zero-calorie sweetener, such as Stevia. When considering tea, the identical principles remain relevant; for your tea to sustain your fasting, it must be of the black variety.

It is equally crucial to acknowledge that any HERBAL INFUSIONS containing FRUIT should be avoided during fasting. Fruits inherently contain glucose, which undoubtedly disrupts the fasting state. Opt for black or green teas instead, as well as spice-infused teas (e.g., Ginger, too, is deemed safe.

What is the mechanism through which coffee and tea suppress appetite? Consuming caffeine has the inherent capacity to induce a sense of satiation or fullness. It additionally facilitates the mobilization of fatty acids within the body, thereby assisting in the transportation of stored fatty acids into the mitochondria, where they are converted into energy, consequently providing an enhanced level of energy. Having increased levels of energy will facilitate the maintenance of optimal levels of productivity and focus during the course of your fast.

Green Tea: Now let us briefly explore green teas. Green tea has the potential to reduce the presence of Ghrelin, the hormone accountable for inducing hunger in our physiological systems. During periods of fasting, it is advisable to infuse green tea in a refrigerated water bottle overnight. (Significant suggestion for achieving leanness) Upon awakening in the morning, consume the entirety of the beverage container prior to breaking your fast. This can enhance your energy levels without experiencing hunger pangs throughout the morning.

4. Experience the benefits of consuming diet sodas with no added sugar, savor the refreshing taste of flavored water without any sugar content, and delight in the chewy satisfaction of sugar-free gum.

To date, there is no substantiated evidence indicating any negative health effects associated with the consumption of artificial sweeteners. Consequently, it would be advisable to consider incorporating these substances into your diet should other methods prove ineffective. It is important, however, to exercise moderation to ensure their impact remains benign.

5. Consider ingesting one or two tablespoons of Psyllium Husk.

Psyllium husk is a fiber supplement that helps massively with hunger, and it signals to your brain that you have food in your digestive system.

6. Cleanse Your Dental Region

This has been empirically demonstrated to diminish the sensation of hunger.

7. Maintain an Active and Dynamic State

Engage in activities that bring you pleasure and fully involve yourself in them, particularly during the early part of the day when your productivity is at its peak.

When one is in a state of flow, time seems to pass quickly, as if 6-7 hours elapse rapidly.

If you are not currently engaged in any additional tasks, it would be beneficial to partake in a brief stroll while simultaneously immersing yourself in an audiobook.

Through this action, you will effectively alleviate excess body fat and acquire further knowledge.

This phenomenon can be characterized as a departure from the norm, as individuals are actively engaging in a state of diminished awareness and mental passivity through their consumption of television and social media.

It is a widely recognized fact that individuals often consume food out of a sense of ennui.

Stay busy, stay productive.

8. Ensure Sufficient Rest

Reduced sleep duration correlates with reductions in leptin levels and increases in ghrelin levels, leading to an augmented sensation of hunger.

A research investigation, juxtaposing two cohorts that adhered to a 700-calorie deficit regimen, while varying the duration of their sleep, yielded the following observations:

The group with a duration of 8.5 hours experienced a roughly equal reduction in both fat and lean mass. The group, which was observed for a period of 5.5 hours, experienced a reduction in both fat and lean mass, with the loss being distributed in a ratio of 20 units of fat to 80 units of lean mass.

Additionally, the study also uncovered that:

If you consistently obtain only six hours of sleep per night for a consecutive period of two weeks, your cognitive and physical abilities deteriorate to an extent comparable to that of staying awake continuously for forty-eight hours.

As is evident, sleep holds utmost importance not only for intermittent fasting but for all aspects of your life.

9. Consume copious amounts of water!

On average, individuals should aim to consume approximately 2 liters of water per day, a quantity that is often not met by most individuals. Adequate hydration is of paramount importance for our bodily functions to operate effectively. When experiencing dehydration, individuals may often experience diminished energy levels, feelings of fatigue, and an increased sensation of hunger. Indeed! It is a well-known fact that our bodies lack a clear signal to indicate the need for water. Instead, we often mistake this need for hunger, even experiencing symptoms such as headaches. Thus, it is essential to prioritize water consumption during fasting periods. Not only can ample water intake help prevent hunger pangs, but it also ensures proper hydration and a sense of well-being. Fasting presents a unique opportunity to diligently monitor and maintain appropriate levels of hydration by closely monitoring our water intake.

10. Carbonated water

Carbonated water can be an excellent aid in alleviating hunger pangs while undertaking a fasting period. Any non-flavored carbonated water or unsweetened carbonated beverages containing zero calories can be consumed without any concerns during periods of fasting (e.g. Le Croix, Bubbly). Carbonated water has the propensity to induce a greater sensation of satiety compared to regular water due to its carbon dioxide content. The rapid inflation of the stomach caused by carbon dioxide can be considerably advantageous in alleviating intense food cravings.

In summary, the matter of hunger experienced during intermittent fasting is merely a temporary concern during the initial weeks until your body acclimates to the altered schedule.

The concepts elucidated herein shall assist you in navigating through challenging circumstances. Currently, the majority of individuals no longer experience hunger after 4-8 weeks of engaging in intermittent fasting. Therefore, it can be confidently asserted that the most challenging timeframe comprises the initial two to three weeks.

Moreover, in the event that significant enhancements are not observed within a duration of four weeks, it is possible that the practice of intermittent fasting may not be suitable for you. Research scientists concur that this approach is not universally applicable for all individuals.

Commencing this diet might appear slightly daunting. Irrespective of the efficacy of this diet in promoting weight loss, the level of intimidation remains unaltered. Prior to embarking on this dietary regimen, it is imperative to grasp that it transcends the conventional notion of a mere diet and encompasses a comprehensive lifestyle approach. Shall we commence the process of formulating a detailed plan in order to facilitate your prompt initiation?

Firstly, choose the fasting technique.

Based on your objectives for achieving weight loss, as well as considering factors such as your preferred lifestyle and individual disposition, you have the option to choose a specific fasting approach. You should select a technique that is compatible with your requirements. Your designated period for nourishment would span from 10 am to 4 pm. If perchance you possess a preference for mornings and derive pleasure from exercising during that time, then selecting the 24-hour fasting regimen would be advisable. Therefore, the eat-stop-eat approach would be the most suitable option for you. If one believes it feasible to abstain from consuming any sustenance throughout the entirety of a day and subsequently partake in a single substantial meal at its conclusion, the warrior diet may be pursued as an alternative.

Second step: Extensive research

It will be necessary for you to conduct extensive research in order to determine the dietary plan that would be most suitable for you. Please carefully review the contents of this book to determine if the dietary plan that best suits your preferences aligns with your lifestyle. Should this be the case, you may choose to adhere to it. Please choose a specific approach that would be suitable for your needs. The nature of your research will be contingent upon the objectives you have established. Prior to commencing, it is advisable to first focus your attention on delineating your objectives. In the event that you express an inclination towards altering your physical composition, specifically by reducing adipose tissue, you may consider adopting the 16/8 method. Regardless of the chosen fasting methodology, it is imperative that the duration of the fasting period does not surpass 72 hours.

Phase 3: Acquiring the essential instruments

Several online applications are accessible that can facilitate your adherence to this dietary regimen. There are complimentary and premium applications available for various mobile platforms.

These applications will assist you in monitoring the progress of your fasting. It is imperative to bear in mind that intermittent fasting entails a process of experimentation and fine tuning. You cannot ascertain the optimal method without firsthand experimentation and experience. These applications will assist you in monitoring your eating and fasting intervals, while also facilitating calorie tracking. As an alternative, you could consistently keep a food diary to monitor and document your progress.

Step 4: The progression

It is a situation where success or failure relies entirely on one outcome. Should you not adopt this particular mindset towards the diet, adhering to it may present challenges. It is possible that you are not accustomed to fasting, and at first, the idea of enduring extended periods of time without consuming food may seem rather daunting. Adjusting to this diet may require some time and effort; nevertheless, it becomes progressively more manageable as one becomes accustomed to it. It is necessary to gradually train your body to adapt to this eating pattern. You may initiate the process by incorporating higher quantities of protein into your dietary intake, while simultaneously reducing the consumption of superfluous sugars and carbohydrates. Consuming protein enhances satiety, enabling one to sustain longer periods without experiencing hunger or craving for food.

Step 5: Establishing a system of support

Having a support system proves to be highly advantageous. It is advantageous to commence this diet alongside a companion. Your choice of a dieting partner may encompass individuals within your social circle, such as a friend, spouse, or family member. You may engage in collective progression through the various phases of the diet, fostering interdependency for mutual encouragement and assistance. In times of discouragement, there will invariably be individuals who can provide the necessary support and guidance to bolster your motivation and ensure your continued progress.

Step 6: Gradually reduce the intensity of your exercise regimen, particularly in the beginning stages.

Usually, potency requires minimalism. Similar to the dissipation of potency observed in alcoholic beverages or coffee when water is added, the effectiveness of your exercise regimen during intermittent fasting would similarly wane if you engage in excessive or excessively intense training. Could you please provide a detailed description of the signs and symptoms that would be indicative of over-training in this particular scenario? A clear illustration would be engaging in protracted periods of exercise characterized by an exceedingly high level of intensity. If you excessively strain yourself, there is a potential for experiencing burnout and subsequently, compromising your health. It is advisable, particularly during the initial phase of this diet, to refrain from engaging in any high-intensity exercise routines. With a progressive enhancement of exercise intensity, your body will gradually acclimate to the dietary regimen.

Excessive training may result in symptoms such as dizziness, fatigue, muscle soreness, and a general sense of weakness. One straightforward examination can be undertaken in order to determine if one is exerting oneself or not. This phenomenon is commonly referred to as the talk test. If one is capable of actively participating in a customary discourse while exercising, albeit with some slight challenge, then it can be classified as moderate. If you exhibit a level of verbal proficiency akin to that which you would employ during an informal conversation with a friend, or if your ability to speak is noticeably impaired, you are experiencing under or over training, correspondingly.

Step 7: Practicing deferred gratification

Exercising patience and postponing immediate satisfaction is an effective strategy. It exhibits remarkable efficacy when paired with intermittent fasting. If your colleagues at your workplace happen to have delectable delicacies, and you find yourself in a state of voracious hunger, your rational mind will likely prompt you to succumb. Upon the onset of hunger, even a serving of cereals adorned with a sprinkling of frost and complemented by a creamy, cool milk appears highly enticing. You must acknowledge that you have the ability to consume everything; however, it is currently not appropriate to do so. You may also choose to document the inventory of foods from which you abstained. This will aid in managing your hunger pangs effectively.

Step 8: Give precedence to protein

It is advisable to consume protein before carbohydrates or any other food items. It may be advisable to consider consuming food items that contain high sugar or fat content, which could potentially pose a significant challenge. If you consume a variety of unhealthy foods, it would render this diet ineffective. You will simply be ingesting an excess of empty calories lacking essential nutrients. It would be beneficial to prearrange your meals and ensure that they contain adequate amounts of protein and complex carbohydrates. It is probable that you will develop an inclination towards these items as your designated eating period draws near. Ensure that you consume grilled chicken, lentils, or an alternative protein source, along with nutritious vegetables. You have the option to incorporate a moderate amount of carbohydrates by including items such as sweet potatoes, potatoes, a portion of rice, or other starchy foods. In light of all that has transpired, there will be no room left for yielding to your desires for unhealthy snacks.

Step 9: Pre-capture image

There is a specific action that you must undertake before commencing with the practice of intermittent fasting. It is advisable that you capture an image of yourself prior to commencing this dietary regimen. Upon commencing the dietary regimen, noticeable improvements in your physique will manifest within the initial fortnight. In addition, it will furnish you with the indispensable impetus to persist. You will have the opportunity to assess your progress by contrasting yourself against that depiction. This will undoubtedly foster a continued desire to persevere. Over time, a noticeable improvement will manifest in your physical being.

Step 10: Considerations to bear in mind

If you are a beginner in adopting this dietary plan, it is important to take into consideration a few factors. The first fortnight poses the greatest challenge, however, subsequent progress becomes increasingly manageable. This current period presents the greatest challenges as your physical constitution adapts to the fasting regimen. Gradually, you will begin to exert authority over your desires, sensations of hunger, and your inclination to eat as well. The adjustment period of your body to the diet can range from several days to several weeks. Therefore, allow yourself an ample amount of time for acclimatizing to the dietary regimen.

When making the decision to incorporate fasting into your lifestyle, it is imperative to ensure the adoption of a health-conscious way of living. This entails incorporating all the components encompassed within this chapter. If you have not already incorporated them, it is advisable to commence their inclusion now. If any of these elements are absent from your life, you will undoubtedly encounter significant challenges when undertaking fasting. Therefore, consider these elements as fundamental prerequisites, as they are inherently indispensable.

Exercise

Our society is predominantly characterized by a high degree of physical inactivity. Hence, a considerable number of individuals encounter difficulties related to their weight and mobility. In my sister's household, as a case in point, both she and my brother-in-law were individuals of above-average weight whose lifestyles were characterized by hectic schedules that did not particularly promote physical activity. The onset of my brother-in-law's mobility issues occurred years ago, prompting them to embark upon a gradual exercise regimen. Initially, they began by leisurely strolling around the neighborhood a few times, gradually elevating their activity level over time. Please refrain from stating that you are unable to accomplish the task. They were perhaps the most physically inept individuals one could envision, and yet they accomplished the task. It is imperative that you relocate the body, as failure to do so may render it subsequently arduous to extricate yourself from your seated position. Despite the inability to engage in strenuous physical activity, it is advisable to commence with modest efforts. Subsequently, they engaged in aquatic activities, thereby facilitating a remarkable form of physical exercise that additionally imparts the art of proper respiration. There exists a wide array of enjoyable exercises that one can engage in. The term "exercise" does not necessarily need to be viewed negatively.

If one possesses a canine companion, it serves as a valid motive to engage in a leisurely stroll outdoors. If one is confined to their residence, they can still engage in physical activity as exercise is a versatile endeavor that can be pursued regardless of location. Moreover, with the proliferation of numerous applications, individuals can even partake in exercise routines within the confines of their personal living space, ensuring utmost privacy. It is important to understand that physical activity facilitates the proper distribution of consumed nutrients throughout the body. In contrast, a sedentary lifestyle characterized by excessive eating without sufficient movement can lead to the accumulation of excess fat.

Water

The consumption of water is imperative for individuals contemplating fasting. It is recommended to consume up to eight glasses of water daily, however, a significant number of individuals fail to adhere to this guideline. Let us now examine the effects of consuming water. Water facilitates the conveyance of nutrients present in foods to various regions of the body. Maintaining proper hydration is essential for your overall well-being. While you may not realize its significance, we aim to demonstrate the consequences of inadequate water intake. The elimination of waste and bacteria from the body is not expedited or facilitated. There exists the potential for the development of diseases such as colon cancer. Additionally, the human body necessitates water to mitigate inflammation, and if one is endeavoring to achieve weight loss through fasting, water is indispensable. In addition to their high water content, uncooked fruits and vegetables possess moisture, thus it is erroneous to assume that hydration can solely be achieved through consumption of water. If you have a genuine intention of employing a detox fasting regimen, the indispensability of water cannot be overstated. Acclimate yourself to consuming water in abundant quantities, but gradually and methodically, as opposed to hastily consuming it in brief intervals. It is imperative to ensure proper hydration by carrying a water bottle at all times during the day. If the taste of water is not appealing, consider incorporating flavorings like a slice of lemon or infusing it with green tea occasionally.

Sleep

It is recommended to obtain a duration of seven to eight hours of sleep per night. In the event that one's health is compromised and they seek to undertake a fasting regimen, it becomes imperative to rely upon the assistance afforded by natural elements. Sleep is a fundamental means through which the body undergoes natural recuperation. Consequently, should one choose to deny themselves sufficient sleep, it is unreasonable to anticipate the ability to sustain a prolonged fasting period, as their endurance will inevitably wane. In addition, during the fasting period, the span of seven to eight hours aids in seamlessly navigating through the fasting phase without conscious contemplation. That is of utmost value if you desire to effectively harness the swiftness to your advantage.

Nutrition

It is logical to infer that if one were to undergo a period of fasting followed by the consumption of fifteen bagels, the weight that was intended to be lost would remain intact. Maintain truthfulness with oneself during the period of fasting. Fasting isn't a fad. It's a lifestyle choice. You have embraced this way of life due to your desire for a more streamlined weight loss experience. While it is true that you possess the permission to indulge in culinary delights, it is of minimal value if one lacks the discernment to make wise dietary decisions. It is imperative to consume a diverse range of fruits and vegetables while exercising moderation in the consumption of high-sugar and trans fatty foods, as excessive intake of such substances can have detrimental effects on one's overall diet.

Is Intermittent Fasting efficacious?

Intermittent fasting aims to create a state in which the body can access stored energy reserves and abstain from food consumption without reaching a condition of starvation. Starvation mode refers to a physiological state in which the body, after enduring extended periods of caloric deficiency, reacts by efficiently conserving any subsequent intake of food energy, swiftly storing it as reserves as a precautionary measure against potential future scarcity. This is the underlying reason for the lack of success observed in the trend of "yo-yo dieting". Individuals subject themselves to states of deprivation, resulting in weight gain upon resumption of regular eating habits. This is similarly why it is crucial to adhere to a suitable fasting regimen, as one should strive to mitigate the occurrence of physiological starvation response.

Scholarly investigation regarding weight reduction has been conducted since the 1920s. Research pertaining to fasting has yielded similar outcomes across a range of subjects, including fruit flies and monkeys. Fasting indeed impacts the composition of what is lost. Majority of dietary approaches lead to reduction in fat, water, and to some extent, muscle. However, intermittent fasting has demonstrated the ability to specifically target and prioritize the loss of fat. It accomplishes this by selecting the optimal energy source during your fasting period. Typically, the human body would preferentially select glucose present in the bloodstream or temporarily stored glycogen in the liver owing to their comparative ease of metabolic processing.

When one engages in fasting, these resources are rendered inaccessible, thereby compelling the body to opt for fat, the sole remaining reservoir of stored energy. This holds particularly true in the context of physical exercise. If you have previously attempted to consume protein shakes prior to exercising and have not observed any notable enhancements, it is because your body is opting to metabolize the shake instead of targeting any surplus body fat you may possess. Engaging in physical exercise while in a state of fasting compels the body to metabolize fat in order to sustain adequate levels of energy.

Whilst in a state of fasting, your body not only triggers the burning of fat reserves, but also heightens its responsiveness to insulin. When contemplating insulin, a prevalent association arises in most individuals - that it is a vital requirement for those afflicted with diabetes. The primary cause for this necessity can be attributed to either the body experiencing a decreased sensitivity towards its own insulin, or a deficient production of insulin. Insulin plays a crucial role in the regulation of blood sugar levels, and individuals who are overweight frequently encounter imbalances in this regard due to the excessive production of insulin, resulting in desensitization of the body to its effects. Fasting can boost sensitivity levels by depriving the body of its usual intake of glucose obtained from frequent eating, thereby enhancing the body's responsiveness.

This tool holds significant value as it facilitates the process of desensitization, wherein your body may opt to store a greater proportion of the glycogen it produces, rather than utilizing it immediately. This mechanism helps stabilize your blood glucose levels, preventing undesirable fluctuations. With the global rise of the obesity problem, there is a corresponding increase in research dedicated to studying dietary phenomena. Fasting is backed by an abundant body of scientific evidence that substantiates its efficacy. What occurs during a day when abstaining from food and drink is not practiced?

Consistently consuming food enables the body to continuously utilize the glucose present in the bloodstream as its primary source of energy. Insulin sensitivity will be within the range of normalcy, although in certain scenarios, it may exhibit signs of desensitization. Glycogen stores that can be readily processed will be replete, leading to surplus energy being efficiently stored as adipose tissue. Consuming a surplus of calories, be it 20 or 200 beyond the required quantity, will result in the accumulation of body fat, as the body does not necessitate the utilization of stored energy.

Fasting can be regarded as a form of training, wherein one endeavors to enhance their body's efficacy in nutrient utilization. The sole reliance on physiological justifications holds significant merit, although it is imperative to consider the additional advantages entailed in weight reduction. Individuals with a lower body weight experience significantly reduced susceptibility to a wide range of health ailments. Moreover, there exists a societal perception of superiority associated with being slimmer, albeit a contentious observation. Additionally, shedding excess weight can yield emotional advantages, promoting an enhanced sense of well-being and contentment in one's life as a whole. Weight loss can additionally result in enhancement across other domains, as individuals with excess weight often experience adverse effects on their knees or back due to the burden of carrying additional body mass.

The aforementioned benefits of fasting are merely the usual ones. One significant aspect of the aforementioned benefits pertains to the notion that each individual who derives advantages from fasting does so due to the conviction that uniqueness is inherent in every person. Surely, every individual undertaking the fast will attain the specific outcome they aspire for.

Intermittent fasting has emerged as a significant trend in contemporary times. Recent reports indicate that individuals who have experimented with such methods have experienced weight loss and improvements in their overall health. Merely to offer you an understanding, intermittent fasting is a dietary approach wherein one is expected to alternate periods of abstinence from food, often consuming only water, while on the other hand, non-fasting refers to the unrestricted ingestion of food, irrespective of its high fat content.

In essence, an individual is able to consume a variety of food items of their choosing over a span of 24 hours, and then abstain from eating for the subsequent 24-hour duration. This approach to weight management is founded on extensive research and adheres to ethical standards upheld globally. When the individual delivers a presentation on intermittent fasting, they will undoubtedly attain their desired outcome.

It is probable that you will observe a wide array of intermittent fasting methods. It can be observed that there are currently two types of intermittent fasting, which are widely practiced and considered the most accessible. First could be the daily fasting in which the person only grows to take in once just about every 20-28 hours within a 4-hour period. The second reason pertains to the practice of fasting intermittently for a duration of 1-3 times per week, commonly known as alternate day fasting. This involves indulging in unrestricted eating on one day, followed by a complete abstinence from food on the subsequent day.

Intermittent fasting has exhibited numerous advantageous impacts when tested on fauna, such as animals and primates alike. A study reveals that individuals who engage in fasting demonstrate a discernible reduction in insulin levels, resulting in an enhanced resistance of neuronal cells in the brain. In 2008, a comprehensive study was conducted on the effects of intermittent fasting, which conclusively demonstrated a significant increase in the average lifespan of individuals by 40.4% and 56.6% in category C. The individuals who engage in intermittent fasting have demonstrated a tendency to shed more weight compared to those following a conventional dietary regimen. In addition, it was demonstrated in a 2009 study that intermittent fasting in rats enhanced their survival rates following sustained heart failure through the promotion of angiogenesis, thereby leading to an extended lifespan for these subjects.

The study merely indicates a concern, namely that there is a limited body of research pertaining to individuals who practice intermittent fasting. The findings pertaining to the higher frequency encompassed within the constitution of the physique and physical activities are intriguing, and remain unexplored within the scholarly circle of your research community. Nevertheless, there exist numerous favorable outcomes. In the preceding month, a study conducted by the National Academy of Sciences published a book that asserts that the act of reducing daily caloric intake by 30% will likely enhance cognitive performance in elderly individuals. In the year 2007, the journal Free Radical Biology & Medicine revealed that individuals suffering from bronchial asthma experienced a notable reduction in symptoms and a corresponding decrease in blood markers as compared to their initial condition.